The Hyperthyroidism Handbook
BY LINDSEY P

An Everyday Guide to Natural Solutions of Living with Hyperthyroidism including Weight Gain, Increased Energy and General Well-being

The Hyperthyroidism Handbook

Copyright 2014 by Lindsey P - All rights reserved.

In no way is it legal to reproduce, duplicate, or transmit any part of this document in either electronic means or in printed format. Recording of this publication is strictly prohibited and any storage of this document is not allowed unless with written permission from the publisher. All rights reserved.

Table of Contents

Introduction 4
Chapter 1: Hyperthyroidism Defined 5
Chapter 2: What are the Causes of Hyperthyroidism? 7
Chapter 3: The Risk Factors for Hyperthyroidism 9
Chapter 4: The Prevention of Hyperthyroidism 13
Chapter 5: Signs and Symptoms of Hyperthyroidism 16
Chapter 6: How Is Hyperthyroidism Diagnosed? 20
Chapter 7: How is Hyperthyroidism Treated? 22
Chapter 8: Thyroid Storm and Hypothyroidism 25
Chapter 9: Managing and Coping with Hyperthyroidism 26
Chapter 10: 10 Natural Home Remedies for Dealing with Hyperthyroidism 30
Chapter 11: Simple Tips for Living with Hyperthyroidism 33
Conclusion 36
Check Out My Other Books 37

Introduction

I want to thank you and congratulate you for purchasing the book, *"The Hyperthyroidism Handbook: An Everyday Guide to Natural Solutions of Living with Hyperthyroidism including Weight Gain, Increased Energy and General Well-being"*.

This book contains proven steps and strategies on how to recognize and diagnose hyperthyroidism based on the signs and symptoms at an early stage to prevent the worsening of the disorder. If in case the disorder has progressed already, this book serves as an ultimate guide on how to live with hyperthyroidism in the best and healthiest possible ways.

Hyperthyroidism is a disease of the thyroid gland. This book is not intended as a medical substitute. It only serves as a guide on how life can be easier for someone who suffers from the disease. Medical help is very important and patients should first seek medical attention.

Comprehensive information on hyperthyroidism is provided on this book. Readers will know how hyperthyroidism is diagnosed, treated and what causes it. Knowledge of the disease should not be limited to doctors alone. It is especially important for the patient and his family members to be knowledgeable about the disease so that they can help the patient avoid the things that should be avoided and pursue all the things that can lead to the betterment of the patient's general health and well-being.

Thanks again for purchasing this book. I hope you enjoy it!

Chapter 1: Hyperthyroidism Defined

Overactive thyroid is also another popular name for hyperthyroidism. This condition is characterized by the excessive production and secretion of the thyroid hormones known as T3 or triiodothyronine and T4 or thyroxine – free hormones secreted by the thyroid gland which are not protein-bound and are released into the blood stream. The most popular cause of this condition is the Grave's disease (which will be further discussed on the causes of hyperthyroidism) and the opposite condition is called the sluggish thyroid otherwise known as the hypothyroidism for it is characterized by a reduction in the production and secretion of the thyroid hormones T3 and T4.

An overactive thyroid is the result of a clinical syndrome known as thyrotoxicosis that occurs when the serum levels of T3 and T4 are unusually high in the bloodstream. Thyrotoxicosis however, can still develop in the absence of hyperthyroidism. When there is an inflamed thyroid gland- a condition known as thyroiditis- thyrotoxicosis occurs as the stored hormones in the swollen thyroid gland are released in excessive amounts even without the production of T3 and T4 which characterizes hyperthyroidism. Furthermore, the condition thyrotoxicosis can develop as a result of too much ingestion of the levothyroxine which is an exogenous thyroid hormone sold in the market as a supplementary thyroid hormone. This phenomenon is clinically dubbed as alimentary thyrotoxicosis, exogenous thyrotoxicosis or occult factitial thyrotoxicosis.

Although hyperthyroidism causes thyrotoxicosis, the therapy and treatment as well as the medical management of the disease is different from the thyrotoxicosis caused by other condition and that which is caused by hyperthyroidism. Different methods are utilized clinically to diagnose and apply appropriate treatments such as radiotracer thyroid measurements and thyroid imaging.

Thyroid Hormones and the Process:

Cell metabolism is stimulated by the thyroid hormones which are produced by the thyroid gland. The thyroid gland is situated below the adam's apple in men and at the lower part of the neck in women and children just above the collar bones. It is shaped like a butterfly complete with the two lobes that form like wings and the isthmus which looks like the body of the butterfly. The thyroid gland envelops the trachea or the wind pipe.

The thyroid gland functions by extracting iodine in the blood which then uses it in the production of the thyroid hormones. Iodine is the primary component needed by the thyroid gland to function normally. It comes from the food we eat like salt, bread and seafood. The 2 most important hormones produced by the thyroid gland are triiodothyronine or T3 and the thyroxine or the T4. 99.9 percent of the hormones produced by the thyroid gland consist of the T4 while .1 percent is T3. Although T3 constitute only .01 % of the hormones produced by the thyroid gland, it is the most active or potent hormone as it has the biggest impact on the body. It has the most biological activity when released in the bloodstream. Since it is more important than the T4, most T4 hormones will then be converted to T-3 when it reaches the bloodstream to complement the necessity for active hormones in the body.

The Process:

There is a chain of command being followed in the regulation of thyroid hormones. It is not surprising because the human body is governed by different internal processes. The thyroid gland is regulated by the pituitary gland, which is another gland located in the brain. Similarly, the pituitary gland is regulated by the thyroid gland in a 'feedback' effect of thyroid hormones in the pituitary. Both glands are then regulated by the hypothalamus, which is another important gland located in the brain.

The hypothalamus releases thyrotropin (TRH) which signals the pituitary gland to release the thyroid-stimulating hormones (TSH). Once TSH is released in the bloodstream, the thyroid gland will then release thyroid hormones which are T3 and T4. If there are any disruptions the supply of the hormones will be reduced causing hypothyroidism. But if there is another condition, like grave's disease, the thyroid gland will release excessive amounts of T3 and T4 resulting to hyperthyroidism.

The pituitary gland controls thyroid hormone production. As a result, if there's insufficient supply of thyroid hormone circulating in the blood stream for normal cell metabolism, the pituitary gland will attempt to balance the insufficiency by producing more thyroid-stimulating hormones (TSH) to stimulate more thyroid hormone production. In contrast, if there's excessive amount of thyroid hormones in the blood, the pituitary gland will decrease the production of TSH to lower the production of thyroid hormones.

Chapter 2: What are the Causes of Hyperthyroidism?

Several factors can cause hyperthyroidism. Oftentimes, when the entire thyroid gland malfunctions it results to the overproduction of thyroid hormones. Excessive secretion of the thyroid hormones may also be a result of a single 'hot' nodule. Thyroiditis which is an inflammation of the thyroid also causes hyperthyroidism. Aside from these causes, there are other clinical conditions that may result to hyperthyroidism. These are the following:

1. **Grave's Disease**: It is an autoimmune disease which may be characterized by different levels of iodine found in the human diet. This phenomenon results to the thyroid's over-activity which then causes hyperthyroidism. A person diagnosed with Grave's disease has a thyroid gland which cannot respond properly to the command or signals sent by the pituitary glands through the secretion of the Thyroid stimulating hormones or TSH. Women are five times more susceptible to this disease than men. It is also hereditary. Diagnosis includes the detection of antibodies like TSI or thyroid stimulating immunoglobulin, TSH receptor antibodies and the thyroid peroxidase antibodies which are believed to be inherent to the disease.

   Grave's disease can be triggered by many factors. These include: radiation to the neck, stress, medications, smoking and viral infections. Standard diagnosis makes use of the nuclear medicine known as thyroid scan/imaging. This method can capture images of the increased levels of the iodine in the blood which are initially labeled with radioactive sensors. Blood test is also used to determine the elevated levels of TSI in the blood.

   Aside from hyperthyroidism, Grave's disease can also cause skin lesions or dermopathy and eye disease known as Grave's ophthalmopathy which can occur on, before or after hyperthyroidism is diagnosed. Ophthalmopathy is characterized by a feeling of sand in the eyes, double vision, sensitivity to light, and protruded eyes. Those who smoke generally experience worse symptoms. In treating ophthalmopathy, surgery may be required as well as steroid therapy to regulate the inflammation. Lastly, dermopathy is quite rare and when it does occur, it is usually painless. The rash is reddish and lumpy and it usually occurs on the frontal area of the legs.

2. **Toxic multinodular goiter and adenoma**: As people age, the thyroid gland becomes naturally lumpy. These lumps are natural and they require no medical attention as they do not produce any thyroid hormones. There are times when a nodule starts to grow bigger than the rest (more than 3cm) and may become autonomous in the process. When a nodule becomes autonomous, it produces hormones independently and does not respond to the signals from the pituitary gland through the thyroid stimulating hormones (TSH). This single nodule may not have any serious impact on the thyroid but when more than one nodule becomes larger and autonomous, the

phenomenon becomes toxic and these functioning nodules are detected by a thyroid scanner.

3. **Thyroiditis**: This is known as the inflammation of the thyroid. There are 2 most popular type of Thyroiditis. One is the Hashimoto's Thyroiditis which is a common condition leading to hypothyroidism and the Subacute Thyroiditis which generally occurs after a viral infection. Subacute Thyroiditis is characterized by a sore throat and painful swallowing coupled with a fever. When touched, the thyroid is tender. Neck pains may be reported as well. Another type of Thyroiditis may develop known as the lymphocytic Thyroiditis where lymphocytes or white blood cells may accumulate in the inflamed gland. When this happens, the thyroid gland becomes 'leaky' resulting to an increased level of hormones in the blood. Lymphocytic Thyroiditis commonly develops after pregnancy and 8 percent after delivery. After delivery, the hyperthyroid stage usually lasts up to 12 weeks and will then be succeeded by hypothyroid phase which lasts up to 6 months. After this phase, the woman goes back to normal thyroid functioning.

4. **Thyroid Hormones excessive intake:** Patients who are taking some oral thyroid hormones usually take in larger doses because their medications are not properly monitored. Some patients fail to make a follow-up with their doctors so they tend to consume excess thyroid hormones as indicated. There are also instances where the patient overindulge and abuse the medication for weight loss purposes.

5. **Intake of Amiodarone:** This drug is quite similar to thyroxin and intake can result to over or under activity of the thyroid.

6. **Postpartum Thyroiditis**: This occurs in women and affects 7% of those who gave birth. PPT starts with the hyperthyroidism phase which lasts up to a few weeks to a few months and then goes back to normal.

7. **Struma Ovarii**: Monodermal teratoma which is rarely detected and contains mostly thyroid tissue that results to hyperthyroidism.

8. **Iodine excessive consumption**: This may be a result of over-eating of foods rich in iodine such as kelp, salt, and other seafood. Similarly, a drug known as amiodarone contain iodine and intake of such can increase the level of iodine in the blood.

9. **Over-secretion of the TSH in the blood**: At least 1 percent of hyperthyroidism cases is caused by an abnormal secretion of the thyroid-stimulating hormone in the blood by the pituitary gland. This happens when there is a tumor in the pituitary gland. More TSH in the blood signals the thyroid gland to release more thyroid hormones that leads to hyperthyroidism. This phenomenon may also be associated with other conditions associated with the pituitary and an endocrinologist typically performs a series of tests to detect the problem.

Chapter 3: TheRisk Factors for Hyperthyroidism

Like most diseases, there are several risk factors that have to be considered when evaluating the likelihood for an individual to develop hyperthyroidism. It is important to know about these risk factors and see whether any of these apply to you because they will help identify the level of risk you have for acquiring the disease, and form there, assist you by indicating what preventive measures you may take to help lessen these risks. To date, scientists and scholars continue to undergo studies to discover any new possible factors that may lead to a heightened risk of developing the thyroid disease.

Below are the factors that have been proven so far to increase the risk of hyperthyroidism.

Personal History

If you have had a thyroid disease in the past and have recovered from it, there still remains a high risk that you may develop a thyroid disease. For instance, if you had a thyroiditis that was caused by an abnormality in your hormone production during pregnancy and then the condition resolved itself, you have a significantly higher risk of developing any thyroid problem again later on in life, even if none of the other risk factors apply to you. Having a personal history of any form of autoimmune disease (e.g. type 1 diabetes) will also affect your risk of developing autoimmune thyroid conditions such as Graves' disease or Hashimoto's disease.

Family History

A person who belongs in a family that has a history of any form and cause of hyperthyroidism are at a very high risk of acquiring the disease as well. In fact, most types of thyroid diseases, whether under hyperthyroidism or hypothyroidism, are hereditary, which means they can be passed on within family members from one generation to another. The risk increases if the relative who has a thyroid disease is a first-degree relative, and the risk goes even higher if the relative was a female (e.g. daughter, sister, and mother). Also, having a relative with autoimmune diseases can elevate risks of you acquiring autoimmune thyroid conditions such as Graves' disease or Hashimoto's disease.

Gender

It has been proven that gender plays a major role in determining the risk of developing hyperthyroidism and other thyroid disorders. Women have a significantly higher risk of developing thyroid diseases when compared to men. Experts have yet to agree on the estimated level of risk increase in women, but it is said by most that women are at risk of developing thyroid disorders around 6 to 8 times more than men. This means that out of 100 patients with thyroid problems, about 60 to 80 of them are women, and the remaining minority are men.

Age

It is possible to develop thyroid diseases at any age, and there are even infants who are born with the condition. However, a young individual who may not have developed a thyroid disease yet can have an increasing risk of developing it as he or she reaches the age of 50. While it can strike at any age, most hyperthyroid (and hypothyroid) diseases develop at 50 and above.

Ethnicity

A number of studies show that people who have a Japanese ancestry have a greater risk of developing hyperthyroid conditions. Experts are still trying to establish the true cause of this, and if there are other ethnicities that contribute to the risk of developing hyperthyroidism. It is said by many, however, that this can be attributed to the fact that Japanese diet is significantly higher than most in the amount of saltwater fish consumed, which increases the amount of iodine intake and consequently increases risk of having an overactive thyroid.

Diet

Diet plays a major role in developing thyroid diseases. Hyperthyroidism can result from too much iodine in the body, so people who observe diets that are high in iodine intake are at a greater risk of developing the disease. This includes iodized and sea salt, sea foods, and some dairy products. Some refined foods, such as refined sugars and pastas, can also increase the risk for hyperthyroidism, as can high-fat cooking oils, trans fatty acids, and most commercially cooked foods and fast foods.

Cigarette Smoking

It has been proven that individuals who are either active or past smokers have a higher risk of developing autoimmune thyroid diseases than non-smokers. This is because cigarettes contain a chemical called thiocyanate, which is an anti-thyroid agent that affects and disrupts the proper function of the thyroid glands. It has also been found that active smoking can worsen the severity and effects of thyroid diseases. Furthermore, it has been found that active smokers are less responsive when it comes to treatments for thyroid diseases that affect the eye, such as Graves' ophthalmopathy.

Medical Conditions

Having other autoimmune diseases can increase an individual's risk of developing autoimmune hyperthyroidism. In some cases, common viral infections can disrupt the thyroid glands and result in a thyroid disease. During and up to a year after pregnancy, a woman is also at a higher risk of developing either a hyperactive or sluggish thyroid, because of how her hormonal production responds to the changes in her body. While most cases of thyroid diseases caused by pregnancy will eventually correct themselves, these women remain at an increased risk of developing a thyroid disease again. Cancers and certain other medical conditions can also lead to thyroid diseases not because of the condition itself but because of the need to undergo radiation exposure treatments, as to be discussed below.

Exposure to Radiation

Individuals who are exposed to radiation, whether accidentally or for the treatment of a medical condition, have a higher risk of developing thyroid cancer and autoimmune thyroid diseases. This is especially true for patients whose neck areas are often exposed to radiation therapy for the treatment of neck or head cancers. An example of accidental radiation exposure is the Chernobyl nuclear accident in1986, after which people were exposed to air, water and food that were contaminated with radiation. Because of the incident, the affected people are at an increased risk of thyroid cancers and other autoimmune thyroid diseases.

Medical Procedures, Supplements, and Medicines

Some individuals who require the intake of herbal supplements and other medications that contain iodine, whether in pill or liquid form, are at a higher risk of autoimmune hyperthyroidism, especially if the individual taking the supplements is already iodine sufficient. There are also certain medical tests and procedures that may expose an individual to more iodine than necessary, such as some tests that use contrast dyes or contrast agents that are iodine-based. Also, most antiseptics used on a person after he or she undergoes surgery (such as Povidone) can slightly increase the individual's risk of developing a temporary thyroid disease.

Neck Trauma or Procedures

A lot of research has gone into the risk of developing thyroid diseases among people who have recently undergone neck, biopsy, surgery , injection in the neck area, or trauma. Usually, thyroid problems that emerge from such incidents are temporary, but there are current debates on the existence of post-traumatic thyroid diseases that occur for a longer term.

Stress

Because stress is considered as an environmental factor that may contribute to the risk of developing autoimmune thyroid diseases, individuals who are going through major life events that may cause major stress (e.g. divorce, death, or physical accidents), may be at a higher risk of acquiring hyperthyroidism.

Left-handedness

While it is not yet considered a definitely established fact, a lot of research points to an increased risk of autoimmune thyroid diseases in left-handed people. The same researches also include people who are ambidextrous and prematurely gray among individuals who have a higher risk in developing the condition, as well as other autoimmune diseases. The theory is that the genetic traits in these people also share a certain gene that is present in most, if not all, autoimmune diseases in general. While the relationship is still under debate, some endocrinologists already factor in these traits when evaluating a patient's risk of developing autoimmune thyroid diseases.

If you have any of the above risk factors, it is best to discuss this with your physician because this means that there is a slightly higher possibility that you might develop hyperthyroidism if you don't already have it yet. The more risk factors apply to you, the higher the possibility that you already have or will develop a hyperthyroid condition.

However, one should note that it is also possible to develop the disease even if none of the abovementioned risk factors apply to him. It is for this reason that it is vital for a person to be aware of the signs and symptoms that may indicate that a person has an overactive thyroid, as to be discussed in the next chapter.

Chapter 4: The Prevention of Hyperthyroidism

In the previous chapter, you learned about the factors that may increase an individual's risk of developing hyperthyroidism. As you may have noticed, a number of these factors cannot exactly be avoided, such as a person's age, gender, ethnicity and personal or family history. A hyperthyroid condition that may result from these factors is often referred to as a "naturally occurring hyperthyroidism," and as such, cannot exactly be prevented.

However, there still is a good possibility that an individual can prevent developing a hyperthyroid condition despite having risk factors that apply to him or her. The first thing to do is to know about what these risk factors are, and then identifying which ones can be managed. Even if an individual may already "have it in his genes," undertaking precautionary measures to prevent the development of hyperthyroidism could still go a long way.

Anti-Hyperthyroidism Diet

An individual's first line of defense in both prevention and cure of *any* medical condition is making the necessary dietary changes. Generally speaking, a diet that seeks to prevent the development of hyperthyroidism in an individual is one that won't increase the body's thyroid hormone levels. Theoretically, this means avoiding foods that are high in iodine, and eating foods that can lower thyroid hormone levels. However, it is important to note that the goal here is to make sure that your thyroid hormone levels remain under control—neither high nor low. Sometimes, when an individual finds that he has a high risk of developing hyperthyroidism, one mistake that he often makes is to research about foods that can quieten the thyroid glands to lower his thyroid hormone levels. These foods are often called goitrogenic foods, such as soy, cabbage, broccoli, cauliflower, spinach, radishes, turnips, kale, millet, kohlrabi, African cassava, Brussels sprouts, as well as all other cruciferous vegetables. The fact that these foods may depress the thyroid glands means that excessive intake may lead to the opposite of hyperthyroidism, which is also something that you have to prevent. The key to a thyroid-friendly diet is in balance. Consult with a professional dietitian to help you determine the necessary dietary changes that you have to observe, especially if you know that you have a risk of developing thyroid diseases.

Body Cleansing Practices

In any prevention and curing program, body cleansing is an essential process that many people undergo. A good dietary plan is already the first step to body cleansing, but other than this, there are also other means that can help improve a body's overall health and prevent the risk of developing certain disease, including thyroid diseases.

Cleansing can help balance the hormonal levels in the body, and with this, help the thyroid function well so that it is neither sluggish nor overactive. There are several cleansing programs that are available for all age groups, some of which you can simply do at home without the help of a professional, others you would have to enroll to. It is also considered a body cleanse for an active smoker to quit smoking. As explained in the previous chapter, quitting the habit will stop a person's exposure to thiocyanate, which is a huge step in trying to manage the risks of acquiring nay thyroid problem if no already exists. Also, you should not underestimate the power of Water Therapy, which remains to be one of the simplest yet most effective body cleansing therapies that can help prevent most diseases.

Regular Physical Activity

Physical activity can do a lot of things that may help prevent thyroid problems from developing. It can help cleanse the body, relieve both physical and emotional stress, and balance bodily functions such as metabolism, in which the thyroid glands are very much involved. Regular workouts such as going to gym, enrolling in martial arts classes, weight-lifting, and other similar activities, may be good choices, but they are not always ideal for everybody, particularly for those who have issues with their schedule and physical capabilities. Regular exercise may come in many forms, and sometimes, they can be simple, everyday things that you can enjoy. Here are some ideas:

- ✓ Jumping in a mini-trampoline
- ✓ Walking or jogging in the neighborhood
- ✓ Talking your pets for a walk
- ✓ Mowing the lawn
- ✓ Fishing, swimming, rowing, scuba diving, snorkeling, surfing, parasailing, wind surfing, and other water sports and activities (motorized or non-motorized)
- ✓ Trekking, mountain climbing, or going on photo safaris
- ✓ Tai Chi, Yoga, and other forms of physical meditations
- ✓ Dancing, Gymnastics, or Aerobics
- ✓ Sexual activity

A Happy Disposition

As mentioned in the previous chapter, major stress can affect an individual's risk of acquiring autoimmune thyroid diseases. Battling stress can help lessen the risk for hyperthyroidism. Also, the cliché "Laughter is the best medicine" may hold true in this case. According to experts, laughter is also a means of providing the body with a natural "inner massage." Not only can it improve your mood, but also help regenerate the body to restore balance.

Stress Management

There are many ways to battle stress. For some people, spiritual therapy is a very effective means for coping with major stressors. Others study how to do self-meditation and hypnotherapy, while there are also those who prefer to do these with the help of professionals. Psychotherapy and regular consultation with psychiatrists can also help a big deal, as can medications that are meant for coping with depression and other psychological problems (If using medications, make sure to inform your physicians about them). There are also those who prefer de-stressing by engaging in activities that they enjoy, or by surrounding themselves with people from whom they can seek emotional support.

Regular Consultation

Whether or not you are at risk of developing hyperthyroidism (or any other disease, for that matter), it is important to set aside time for undergoing regular check-ups with your physician. Get blood tests periodically so you and your doctor can monitor your thyroid hormone levels. Also make sure that you inform your physician of all supplements and medications that you take, especially if you have another medical condition that you are trying to cure or manage. Both deficiencies and excesses in vitamin and mineral intake can lead to various medical conditions. Make sure that you collaborate with your physician so that you can be certain that the key nutrients in your body, especially iodine in this case, remain balanced.

Knowledge will be your best ally when it comes to preventing the risks of developing hyperthyroidism. The first step is to know about the risk factors so you can easily identify which necessary preventive measures you have to make. Of course, it is always best to do these with the advice of a professional health worker, so that you can be certain not only that your efforts won't go to waste, but also that they won't worsen the odds of you developing a thyroid disease.

It is important to note, however, that these are not cures for hyperthyroidism or any other form of thyroid disease. These are also not fool proof means for dodging hyperthyroidism, especially since some cases are naturally occurring.

Nevertheless, you can never be too careful for as long as your health is concerned. There is no harm in taking preventive measures that you know can greatly reduce the risk of developing a thyroid disease, whether it is a hyperthyroid or hypothyroid condition.

Chapter 5: Signs and Symptoms of Hyperthyroidism

Medically speaking hyperthyroidism is characterized by excessive thyroid hormones in the bloodstream. Physiologically, thyroid hormones play a very important role in the metabolic processes that govern the cellular functions. They affect nearly all types of body tissues. They serve to control the physiological processes in the body otherwise known as the metabolic rate.

Consequently, the amount of thyroid hormones dictates the pace of these metabolic processes. The more thyroid hormones in the blood the faster the processes can become. This is precisely the reason why patients who have hyperthyroidism experience a number of the following symptoms of:

- Irritability
- Nervousness
- Increased heart rate
- Increased perspiration
- Anxiety
- Sleeping difficulties
- Hand tremors
- Fine and brittle hair
- Skin-thinning
- Muscular weaknesses in the areas of the thigh and upper arms
- Weight loss despite good appetite
- Hair loss (outer third of the eyebrows)
- Intolerance to heat
- Fatigue
- General weakness
- Muscle aches
- Hyperglycemia
- Irritability

- Hyperactivity
- Delirium
- Myxedema (in case of Grave's disease)
- Polyuria
- Pretibial
- Difficulty to concentrate
- Panic attacks
- Memory problems.

Diarrhea is reported to be uncommon but frequent bowel movement is more likely. Despite good appetite, considerable weight loss is detected although 10% are more likely to gain weight. Vomiting also is included and women may experience abnormalities in their menstrual flow such as period becoming less frequent or flows may be less heavy.

Increased levels of thyroid hormones in the blood also cause palpitations and increased heart rate similar to that of epinephrine overdose. Other symptoms include: anxiety, hand tremors, hyper-motility of the digestive system, low serum cholesterol and unintended weight loss.

In case of a thyroid storm, the patient experiences paranoia and psychosis but these are less common in cases of hyperthyroidism. Complete reduction of the symptoms is commonly experienced by many during 1-2 months after the period of euthyroid is obtained. Physical symptoms include:

- Shortness of breath
- Loss of libido
- Palpitations
- Vomiting
- Nausea
- Feminization
- Diarrhea.

If left untreated for long-term, hyperthyroidism may lead to osteoporosis.

There were also a number of neurological signs and symptoms established. These include: periodic paralysis (more common in people with Asian descent), tremors, myopathy and chorea. Myasthenia Gravis and hyperthyroidism has also been found to be quite connected. 5% of myasthenic patients have hyperthyroidism. Even after thyroid treatment, myasthenia cannot be cured because it is auto-immune.

As the most common cause of hyperthyroidism, Graves' disease presents other underlying symptoms. Some patients may have goiter due to enlarged thyroid gland. Another common problem caused by Graves' disease includes the enlargement of the eyes due to the swelling of eye muscles, a condition known as Graves' ophthalmopathy. This can happen any time before, at the same time as, or after other symptoms of hyperthyroidism manifest. Patients who experience this may have the following symptoms:

- Eyeball/s sticking out farther than normal
- Bug-eyed or staring look
- Dry, itchy and irritated eyes
- Sensitivity to light
- Teary eyes
- Difficulty in closing the eyes completely, especially when asleep
- A sensation of pain or pressure around the eyes
- Double vision, especially when looking to the sides

Often, mild cases of Graves' ophthalmopathy resolve themselves in around 1 to 4 months' time. These symptoms can be treated with surgical procedures or by taking anti-thyroid medications. If diagnosed in its early stages, it can also be treated with non-steroidal anti-inflammatory drugs or NSAIDs (e.g. naproxen, ibuprofen, aspirin).

Other minor ocular symptoms of hyperthyroidism include: lid-lag, eyelid retraction and extra-ocular muscle weakness. Dalrymple sign or hyperthyroid stare, the eyelids are abnormally retracted upward. Extra-ocular muscle weakness results to double vision. In patients with lid-lag symptoms, the eyelids fail to follow the directions taken by the iris especially when the iris goes downward following a moving object. This is temporary though, and will eventually disappear after treatment.

In a small number of cases, some hyperthyroid patients experience a symptom in which there is an inflammation of the tissues around their eyes. This is called an acute inflammatory thyroid eye disease. People with this symptom will experience:

- Swelling of tissues around the eyes, especially in the morning
- Swelling of the eyelids, especially in the morning
- Swelling of protective membrane covering the eye balls

- A sensation of pain when moving the eyes.

Surgery is rarely used to treat patients with acute inflammatory thyroid disease; doctors usually only resort to surgery if the inflammation is very severe, and if the patient wants his or her eyes to look a bit differently. Like Graves' ophthalmopathy, the inflammation of the tissues around the eyes often simply goes away by themselves after some time. If the inflammation is more severe and doesn't seem to improve on its own, doctors may prescribe the use of immunosuppressants, corticosteroid medications, or radiation therapy.

Lastly, Grave's disease comes with exophthalmos or protrusion of the eyelids. Exophthalmos occurs exclusively to hyperthyroidism caused by Grave's disease although not all exophthalmic symptoms are diagnostic of Grave's disease. With hyperthyroidism, the immune-mediated swelling of the retro-orbital socket (eye socket) causes the eyes to protrude.

Chapter 6: How is Hyperthyroidism Diagnosed?

When hyperthyroidism is suspected, the initial test will be the measurement of the TSH (thyroid-stimulating hormones) in the blood. If the TSH level is low, this is an indication that the pituitary gland is signaled by the brain (hypothalamus) to reduce the secretion of the hormones as it detected an increased level of T3 and T4 in the blood. In other occasions, low levels of TSH in the blood are indicative of pituitary malfunction or temporary reticence of the pituitary gland due to other medical conditions. This is why TSH measurement is the most important first step to consider.

Diagnosis may also be contributed by the measurement of antibodies associated with the thyroid gland such as anti-TSH receptor antibodies (commonly found in Grave's disease) and the anti-thyroid peroxidase (indicative of Hashimoto's Thyroiditis).

Such diagnosis will only be confirmed when the blood test shows that there is indeed an increased level of T3 and T4 in the blood as well as the reduced level of TSH in the blood. The pituitary gland regulates the amount of thyroid hormones released by the thyroid gland. If there's too much thyroid hormone, the pituitary gland will reduce the level of TSH in the blood instructing the thyroid gland to reduce the thyroid hormones production. The cause of hyperthyroidism can be diagnosed using the thyroid scan as well as the radioactive iodine uptake. The uptake test utilizes radioactive iodine which may be taken orally or injected on an empty stomach to come up with the measurement of iodine being absorbed by the thyroid gland. If the iodine absorption is too much, this means the person has hyperthyroidism. Thyroid scans allow the radiologists and endocrinologists to have a visual examination of the overactive thyroid.

To differentiate hyperthyroidism from Thyroiditis, a method known as scintigraphy is used. There will be two tests connected to each other including the uptake test and the thyroid imaging with the use of gamma camera. Uptake test, as mentioned before uses radioactive iodine (iodine-123 is the most commonly preferred radionuclide but iodine-131 is the traditional radionuclide being used). Iodine-123 is the perfect isotope of iodine for the thyroid tissue imaging and thyroid cancer metastasis.

The administration of this radioactive iodine involves oral consumption of a pill or liquid which contains sodium iodide (NaI) consisting of a small amount of iodine-123. The patient is required to fast for 2 hours prior and 1 hour after the pill ingestion. This method is safe unless the patient has allergic reactions to iodine. The excess radioiodine which was not absorbed by the thyroid gland will then be excreted from the body through urinating. If an allergic reaction occurs, the patient will be given an antihistamine.

After 24 hours, the patient is expected to return for the uptake test. This method utilizes a device with a metal bar placed against the neck that can measure the emitted radioactivity by the thyroid gland. The test takes only 4 minutes until the percentage of the uptake is accumulated and measured by the software. Simultaneous scanning is also taking place where imaging is derived including the left, right and central angle with a gamma camera. The radiologists will be the one to read and interpret the imaging and the report will be filed including the uptake examination results and comments about the imaging. Radioactive iodine intake is usually higher in patients with hyperthyroidism.

Lastly, other doctors test the T3, free T3, T4 and/or Free T4 to come up with better and more accurate results. If the T3 and T4 levels are higher than normal in the blood that indicates that the person has hyperthyroidism.

Chapter 7: How is Hyperthyroidism Treated?

Hyperthyroidism cases typically require an initial treatment using the anti-thyroid drugs or medically known as the suppressive thyrostatics medication. Use of anti-thyroid drugs is temporary. At a more advanced stage, however, radioisotope therapy or surgical procedure may be conducted to permanently resolve hyperthyroidism issues. Unfortunately, all these treatments may cause the thyroid gland to become underactive leading to the opposite condition known as hypothyroidism. When that happens, triiodothyronine and levothyroxine may be taken as supplements to manage the side effects. Surgical options are necessary especially when the thyroid gland is enlarged and may be posing some threats to underlying tissues due to the neck compression structures or when hyperthyroidism is triggered as an effect of a more cancerous origin.

Here are the treatments used to combat hyperthyroidism:

1. **Anti-thyroid drugs**: These are drugs that are powerful enough to reduce the production of thyroid hormones. Examples of these drugs are: propylthiouracil, methimazole (sold in the US) and carbimazole (sold in the UK). These anti-thyroid drugs work by slowing down the iodination of thyroglobulin and in effect will reduce the production of T4 or tetraiodothyronine. Propylthiouracil, on the other hand, prevents the conversion of T4 to T3 outside the thyroid gland when it reaches the bloodstream. It is important to note though, anti-thyroid drugs take effect after a few weeks because of the substantial amount of thyroid hormone stored in the thyroid tissue. The dosage need to be carefully monitored for a period of one month coupled with doctor follow-up and blood tests.

   Initially, a high dose is recommended but if it persisted, hypothyroidism may develop as a result. Block and replace method is also administered to patients where they will be given sufficient dosage of anti-thyroid drugs to block the hormone production completely and then the patients will be treated as hypothyroidism patients.

2. **Food and Diet**: Hyperthyroidism patients cannot be given foods rich in iodine such as kelps and seaweeds. Iodized salts are also believed to have no desired effect but instead it has increased the number of deaths in the United States so that has to be eliminated in the case of hyperthyroidism patients.

3. **Beta-Blockers**: Since hyperthyroidism affects nearly all processes in the body and resulting oftentimes to increased heart rate, palpitations, sweating and the likes, beta-blockers are recommended to tame these symptoms and help the patient to calm down. They regulate the heart beat and minimize the onset of palpitations, hand tremors and anxiety. Beta-blockers offer temporary relief from these symptoms until the procedure of the radioiodine

is administered. They do not treat and therefore cannot be used to treat hyperthyroidism. They can only reduce the symptoms.

Propranolol can also be used to minimize the onset of symptoms. L-propranolol treats the symptoms associated with the nerves such as tremors, anxiety, palpitations and heat intolerance. D-propranolol, on the other hand, blocks the conversion of T4 to T3. Propanolol is most commonly used in the UK while metoprolol is used in the US but both are helpful in treating hyperthyroid patients' symptoms.

4. **Surgery**: Thyroidectomy is a surgical procedure that refers to removing the thyroid gland whether the entire gland or just a part of it. Surgery is the last method used when all else failed but most often, cases are treated and resolved by just administering the radioactive iodine method. Surgical procedures are more complicated because it involves the removal of the parathyroid glands and cutting of the laryngeal nerve resulting to a difficulty in swallowing. There may also be an increased risk of acquiring staphylococcal infection as with any major surgeries. In case of Grave's disease where patients are unable to tolerate the medication and/or allergic to medication especially the radioiodine, surgical procedures are obtained.

5. **Radioiodine**: This is also known as iodine-131 isotope therapy pioneered by Dr. Saul Hertz where the patient is given the radioactive iodine in the form of a pill or liquid which they will have to take in orally. Such method is used once to severely disrupt or completely ruin the function of a hyperactive thyroid gland. Iodine-131 is potentially more potent than iodine-123 (which has a biological half-life from 8-13 hours) for it has a biological half life of up to 8 days. Iodine-131 emits beta particles which are more extremely damaging to the tissues at short range. Once the radioiodine or iodine-131 is administered, the cells will absorb it resulting to their destruction which will eventually render the thyroid gland mostly if not completely inactive.

There are no side effects to this kind of therapy as the destruction is local. Iodine is easily absorbed by the thyroid cells especially the cells of the hyperactive thyroid. It has been constantly used for 50 years since it has started and the only restrictions include pregnancy and breastfeeding as the breast tissues also pick up iodine). After radioiodine therapy, the patient will then be given the supplemental thyroid hormones to complement the body's requirement. A medical report suggests however, that there's a bigger risk of cancer incidents in patients after the radioiodine therapy.

Radioiodine treatment has a bigger chance of success than ordinary medications. The success rate differs and is dependent on the dosage administered and the cause of hyperthyroidism but generally the success rate is between 75-100 percent. In patients suffering from Grave's disease, the major side-effect of the radioiodine treatment is the occurrence of the life-long hypothyroidism which requires a daily treatment or intake of thyroid hormone. Those with eye disease also experience worsening of the condition after the radioiodine treatment. This is one of the reasons why some patients prefer to have the surgical treatment. In other situations where the patient has a different type of disease, or a larger thyroid gland, or if the first treatment did not take effect, the patient may be given another radioactive treatment. It is not surprising to know that many patients feel unhappy about the idea of taking thyroid hormones for the rest of their lives. Even so, thyroid hormones are generally safe, easy to consume, inexpensive, and very much similar to the thyroid hormone created by the thyroid.

It is quite normal for patients who have undergone radioiodine treatment to experience a worsening effect of the hyperthyroidism symptoms for a few weeks to a few months. This is the result of the total destruction of the thyroid tissue where thyroid hormones are released into the blood as thyroid cells containing these hormones are destroyed as well. If this happens, beta-blockers can definitely reduce the symptoms and make it more tolerable for a period of time.

Majority of the patients do not however, encounter any other problems. Some only complain of a little soreness in the throat area or tenderness of the neck but after a few days it will just disappear without any other associated symptoms.

In case of lactating mothers, it is not advised for them to continue breastfeeding for at least a week as radioiodine may still be present in the milk even after the radioiodine treatment.

78 percent of people treated with radioiodine that has Grave's disease develop hypothyroidism and 40 percent of those who have goiter or toxic multinodular goiter and adenoma swing to sluggish thyroid gland condition. To reduce the rate of failure, it is recommended that dosage should be increased for a more potent effect.

Chapter 8: Thyroid Storm and Hypothyroidism

Other conditions that may have a significant connection with hyperthyroidism are thyroid storm and hypothyroidism. Thyroid storm is a condition where hyperthyroidism symptoms occur at the extremes. Aggressive treatment of resuscitation including a combination of the treatments mentioned above plus an intravenous administration of beta-blockers (such as propranolol, succeeded by thioamide (methimazole)) and an iodine solution or iodinated radio contrast agent plus a steroid known as hydrocortisone is administered intravenously.

Thyroid storm is a severe form of hyperthyroidism associated with irregular heartbeats, diarrhea, vomiting, high temperature and mental agitation. It is a medical emergency where hospital treatments and care facilities are required as it is potentially fatal.

Hypothyroidism, on the other hand is the opposite condition of hyperthyroidism, which means that a hypothyroid patient is one whose thyroid hormone levels are below normal. While hyperthyroidism is known to be the result of an overactive thyroid, hypothyroidism occurs when the thyroids shuts down and doesn't produce thyroid hormones or when it can only produce hormones that are way beyond what the body needs for them to perform their metabolic functions properly. This is why where hyperthyroid patients often lose weight despite a good appetite, hypothyroid patients often experience uncontrollable weight gain.

Hypothyroidism is closely connected to hyperthyroidism because most often, people who have been treated with radioiodine develop hypothyroidism as a side effect to the treatment. It is quite expected as the thyroid gland is damaged. It is also not uncommon for hypothyroidism to occur after a hyperthyroid period as the thyroid glands try to make one last attempt to properly function before finally shutting down.

Hypothyroidism cases that result from hyperthyroidism are not at all difficult to manage, and most endocrinologists will agree that they are easier to treat than hyperthyroidism. Nonetheless, a hypothyroidism case has to be given the proper medical attention so that it doesn't worsen. To treat this condition, a regular intake of thyroid hormone is often enough. However, this must only be done with the advice of a physician because taking the wrong amount of thyroid hormones may either not resolve the hypothyroidism, or result in going back to a hyperthyroid state if taken in excess.

Chapter 9: Managing and Coping with Hyperthyroidism

Professional Health Care

It is extremely important for hyperthyroid patients to receive proper and adequate medical care. This means consulting with a physician from diagnosis to treatment and management of your hyperthyroid condition. It is never safe to simply make self-assumptions on whether you have a thyroid disease and what type of thyroid disease you may have. Even more dangerous is any attempt to undergo any form of treatment or take any medications that are meant for hyperthyroid patients without first seeking the advice of your endocrinologist. Taking the wrong types and amount of medications may worsen your condition, cause you to develop new diseases that you didn't have on the onset, and can even be fatal.

It is essential for you to ask questions when there is anything that isn't clear to you about your thyroid disease and the other implications it may have to your overall health. Your medication will be very important in treating your hyperthyroidism, but this isn't the only one that matters. Just as important is the need for you and your physician to regularly monitor your body's thyroid hormone levels. As you take your medications and as your body responds to them, there may be changes in your thyroid hormone levels, and as such, your physician might recommend changes in your medications or dosages. This is to make sure that you maintain balance in the amount of thyroid hormones produced by your glands, so that you neither remain in a hyperthyroid state nor fall into a hypothyroid state as a result of lowering your thyroid hormone levels. Your doctor will help you achieve this balance, so make sure that you consult with him every time you notice any changes in your body and condition, as well as if you have any plans to incorporate other methods for helping you manage your hyperthyroidism, such as the ones listed below.

Hyperthyroidism Diet

Many experts will agree that medications will sometimes be useless if your diet doesn't support the right types and amount of nutrients that is appropriate for addressing your medical condition.

There are several nutritional concepts that you have to be familiar with when it comes to managing your hyperthyroid condition. In general, the idea is to increase your intake of protein, iron, vitamin B, and vitamin D. Also, you will be advised to either avoid or simply regulate your consumption of foods that speed up metabolism, such as coffee, chocolate, black tea, sodas, and foods that are high in iodine. You may also be advised to eat foods that can help suppress the thyroid function, such as soya products and cruciferous vegetables. However, the key is to balance the nutrients that your body needs and not to end up having an excess or deficiency in any if the key nutrients that help in maintaining a balanced and well-functioning thyroid. While there are available guides online, it is still wisest to do this with the help of a dietitian who can make the suitable recommendations based on your thyroid function test results.

Natural Remedies

Besides prescription medicines and a hyperthyroid-friendly diet, many people also rely on natural, alternative remedies for helping them cope with their condition. In some cases, particularly in hyperthyroid diseases that are mild or diagnosed in their early stages, these natural remedies are able to resolve the symptoms and the disease without the patient having to take any prescription medicines. In other cases, a patient still has to take his or her medications and then incorporate these natural home remedies to help relieve the symptoms and even speed up their recovery.

Some of the most popular alternative home remedies involve drinking one to three cups of tea using certain herbs. Examples of these herbs are lemon balm, bugleweed, and motherwort. The next chapter will go into more a detailed explanation of the different safe, easy and effective natural home remedies that are perfect for hyperthyroid patients.

Regular Exercise

Regular physical activity will play a huge role in preventing your condition from worsening, avoiding any other complications and diseases, and keep your hyperthyroidism under control. It can also help regulate certain symptoms that are associated with hyperthyroidism, including anxiety and sleep disturbances.

More importantly, regular physical activity will have a positive impact on a person's weight and metabolism, which are both affected when the thyroid glands do not function well. It also helps improve a hyperthyroid patient's fatigue levels, and there have been several studies that prove that significantly more patients who have Graves' disease can successfully stop their medications and not go through a relapse if they undergo a structured exercise program.

For those who do not have the time to enroll in such exercise programs, there are other alternatives.

Other Lifestyle Changes

There are also some lifestyle changes that you may want to take into consideration if you wish to control the symptoms of your hyperthyroidism and aid in your speedy recovery. Incorporating a healthier diet, good sleeping habits, and regular exercise are already major steps in adapting a healthier lifestyle.

Aside from these, one major factor that you want to put much emphasis into is cigarette smoking. It is near impossible to control your thyroid disease and its symptoms if you are an active smoker.

There are also some environmental toxins that can worsen your condition, so it is best to minimize your exposure to them. With the thousands of chemicals being manufactured and produced by different industrial companies, it is almost impossible to simply choose to live in an area where you can be certain of the air you breathe. However, it is still possible to cut down on the toxins you expose yourself and your family to simply by making better choices when shopping for household products. While it is true that natural household products can be more a bit costly, you can be assured that these will help not only in managing your hyperthyroidism, but in helping improve your overall heath as well.

Stress Management

It is important for an individual with hyperthyroidism to learn how to relax so that he reaches a state of mental calmness. Having a happy, calm and relaxed disposition is not only an attitude or trait that you have to be born with. In fact, it is a learnable skill that you can master with the help of a professional or even by yourself.

It has been well-documented that many thyroid diseases, particular Graves' disease, can be caused by stress, and that their symptoms may also worsen if the patient doesn't know how to handle his or her major stressors.

The simplest yet most effective form of stress management is getting adequate sleep. Adequate doesn't simply mean getting 4 or 5 hours of sleep at night, which may be just "enough" to get by the next day. Sufficient sleep is anywhere between 7 to 8 hours each night. It is also important that you maintain a regular sleep cycle, as your thyroid glands, along with the other glands and organs in your body, also go to a relaxed state whenever you sleep. This will help in regulating your thyroid functions. Also, poor sleeping habits (i.e. lack of sleep, irregular sleeping hours) can have many adverse effects to your adrenal glands and your endocrinal system as a whole.

Aside from sleeping, relaxation and stress management may come in many forms of activities that vary from one person to another. It can be something as simple as listening to music, soaking in a bubble bath, reading a good book in your favorite quiet spot, tending to your garden, taking a stroll in the woods or in the park, just driving around the neighborhood, painting or writing, or even just lying down and letting your body and mind relax. Other people prefer doing more physically extreme activities such as working out in the gym, engaging in different sport activities, doing yoga, Pilates, or Tai Chi, going for a swim, scuba diving or doing any water sports, mountain climbing, hiking, or even doing extreme sports such as sky diving or bungee jumping.

The kind of activities for relaxation for you will depend on several factors such as your preferences, budget, and time constraints. If you do not know what activities are more suitable for you and the kind of lifestyle that you lead, you can ask for the advice of people you know, and you can also discuss this with a therapist who can help you manage your stress.

Continuous Self-Education

Finally, it is important that you keep yourself updated on new studies that are related to your condition. There are still several studies that are going on when it comes to the different causes, risk factors, preventive measures, diagnosis, treatment, and management of hyperthyroidism. The Internet has made it easier for anyone to have quick access to all the latest information and breakthroughs in medicine, and it is important that you take advantage of this. Remember that managing your thyroid disease is not simply a matter of relying on your doctors for information on the things you have to do and avoid doing. You should also try ot help yourself by staying well-informed about your condition so that you can adjust to any new findings related to hyperthyroidism.

Professional health care will indeed play a very important role in helping you cope with your hyperthyroidism. But you should be aware that there's more to the management of this diseases than that.

Managing and coping with hyperthyroidism is more than just about the professional help you get, but also about what you eat and don't eat, what you do and which habits you stop, what you think and what information and new knowledge you continuously allow yourself to learn. Sometimes, it is the small things that you may not notice that can actually make greater impacts in helping you cope with your condition, and even recover from it completely.

Chapter 10: 10 Natural Home Remedies for Dealing with Hyperthyroidism

Aside from medications, surgeries and other medically accepted treatment methods, some people like to rely on natural methods for treating their illnesses.

Hyperthyroid patients are not exempt from this practice. While none of these methods are technically accepted to be actual cures for hyperthyroidism, these natural home remedies have been acknowledged by many patients and doctors alike in helping resolve diseases that develop from overactive thyroid glands. The best thing about them is that they are safe and easy to do.

Below are the 10 most popular all-natural remedies that you can whip up at home to help you manage your hyperthyroid condition.

1. **Lemon Balm** – Also known as Melissa officinalis, Lemon balm is one of the more popular herbal remedies recommended for hyperthyroid individuals. The herb helps bring an overactive thyroid back to a normal state by lowering TSH levels. It also has several useful compounds such as phenolic acids and flavonoids which can help regulate the thyroid glands. Furthermore, the herb blocks antibodies from stimulating the thyroid glands, which can help prevent Graves' disease or cure it if the condition already exists. Patients are advised to drink a cup of lemon balm tea two to three times a day to restore the thyroid glands to their normal state. Some patients prefer to start with a lower dosage of about ½ to 1 teaspoon of lemon balm steeped in a cup of boiling water before gradually increasing to the recommended 2 tablespoons of lemon balm per cup of tea.

2. **Bugleweed** – Also known as Lycopusvirginica, Bugleweed is an herb that is widely recognized to be helpful in managing various hyperthyroid conditions and their symptoms. It works by reducing the hormones secreted by the thyroid glands to normalize thyroid hormone levels. It has been shown to decrease TSH levels in the body, lowers T4 levels, and blocks T4 from converting to T3. It can be taken in tinctures of two to six mL daily. Alternatively, you can also create a Bugleweed tea by steeping ½ teaspoon of the herb in a cup of boiling water then straining the tea to discard the used herbs. Doing this once daily can already help a lot, especially if done in combination with other natural remedies.

3. **Motherwort** – Another herbal remedy that can be consumed in the form of a tea, motherwort is also known as Leonurus cardiac, and can help in managing certain symptoms of hyperthyroidism such as tachycardia and palpitations. It is also known to be a natural beta-blocker and can perform some anti-thyroid activities that will help depress the activity of an overactive thyroid. The recommended dosage for this remedy is ½ teaspoon of motherwort steeped in a cup of boiling water, taken two to three times a day.

It is important to note, however, that motherwort should not be taken if you are on any sedating medications.

4. **Eleuthero** – This herb is important in helping strengthen a person's adrenal glands. While this is not considered a direct remedy for hyperthyroidism, it is in fact important to make sure that the body's entire endocrine system is healthy, starting from the adrenal glands. This can help prevent a person from acquiring autoimmune thyroid problems, as well as help remedy symptoms from conditions such as Graves' disease. Similar to the first three herbs, this can be taken in the form of a cup of tea. Simply steep ½ tsp of the herb in a cup of boiling water, and drink the tea one to two times a day.

5. **Broccoli and Cabbage** – these are cruciferous vegetables that contain a substance known as goitrogen. Goitrogens restrain the overactive thyroid glands from producing too much hormones than necessary, thus normalizing the body's thyroid hormone levels. These foods re best consumed uncooked, as the goitrogens are greater and more effective in that state. Other goitrogenic vegetables include cauliflower, rutabaga, kale, mustard greens, spinach, Brussels sprouts, kohlrabi, turnips, and radishes.

6. **Soy Products** – Soy is also considered a goitrogen, and as such can help in regulating the hormones produced by the thyroid glands. Eating protein-based and more soy products can help improve and treat hyperthyroid conditions.

7. **Indian Gooseberry** – Indian gooseberry can help in treating various medical conditions, hyperthyroidism included. It has ameliorating effects on the thyroid glands that can help regulate the production of hormones to restore balance. You can take fresh Indian gooseberry or simply purchase Indian gooseberry powder from the market. Mix with honey to produce a thick paste that you can eat once daily, preferably in the morning before you take your breakfast.

8. **Berries** – Berries are a very good source of vitamins and minerals. They also have various antioxidant properties, which can help in reducing any inflammation of the thyroid glands and other parts of the body that may have swollen due to the hyperthyroid condition. Simply add different types of berries to your diet (strawberries, blueberries, blackberries, cherries, etc.), and you can eat them as substitute for snacks and desserts.

9. **Sea vegetables** – Contrary to what some people might think, hyperthyroidism doesn't mean completely avoiding any sources of iodine. In fact, due to this wrong notion, many people who are diagnosed with hyperthyroidism eventually develop iodine deficiency, which is also not good for thyroid health. It is still important to eat good, natural sources of iodine, such as kelp, sea palm, nori, and other sea vegetables. Aside from being a good source of iodine, they also have a good amount of magnesium, calcium, iron, folate, and vitamin K. Of course, it is wiser to go through an iodine

loading test to determine your body's iodine level, and from there seek advice on the amount of iodine you should incorporate in your diet.

10. **Omega-3 Fatty Acids** – A body that doesn't have enough Omega-3 fatty acids can go through hormonal imbalance. This includes abnormal levels of thyroid hormones, which can lead to either hyperthyroidism or hypothyroidism. These fatty acids are essential for a number of things, including building hormones that are responsible for controlling cell growth and immune functions, as well as for helping the body respond to thyroid hormones and use them for proper metabolism. Adding more fish, walnuts, flaxseeds, and grass-fed animal products to your diet will increase the amount of omega-3 fatty acids in your body.

For most people, the first three natural remedies mentioned above are the most effective. According to many accounts from people with hyperthyroidism, their conditions either improved or were thoroughly cured by using a combination of lemon balm, bugleweed, and motherwort. They have found that using only one remedy will help a lot, but there are still some symptoms that remain. Incorporating these three remedies has proven to be more effective in many cases, and others also decide to integrate some of the other remedies listed above to help speed up their recovery.

For mild conditions, these natural remedies, coupled with a healthy lifestyle (i.e. good diet, regular exercise, and a sound psychological condition) can often be enough to cure the thyroid disease. However, for more severe cases, it is best to work with your physician in determining which natural methods can be taken with your prescribed medications.

Chapter 11: Simple Tips for Living with Hyperthyroidism

In some cases, hyperthyroidism takes a while before it is treated. In worse cases, the conditions can also be untreatable, and patients are faced with having to live with the condition all their lives. Whichever the case is, patients are often disheartened and worried about not being able to live a normal life anymore.

But unlike other diseases, living with hyperthyroidism isn't as hard to manage. The symptoms aren't as severe, and treating it is often neither painful nor difficult to do. Many people who have hyperthyroidism can still manage to live normal lives even if their condition is untreatable. As long as they continue to follow their doctors' advice on the necessary medications, dietary changes, and physical activities, living with hyperthyroidism is just like living a normal life.

Tips for Living with Hyperthyroidism

1. If you have been advised to take any anti-thyroid medications, make sure that you take them at the same time every day. This will help your thyroid glands adjust to the medications so that they can balance their functions and aren't suddenly disrupted due to an irregular schedule of medicine intake. You can set your alarm so you can be sure that you take them at the same time each day.

2. Make sure that you don't skip on your medications. Again, setting your alarm to remind you of this will come in handy. It is also helpful to have someone at home who can remind you every day about your meds, or to have a medicine box labelled with the days of the week so you can keep track of your medications and be sure that you haven't skipped on any of them.

3. Keep a personal log book in which you can record the results of your thyroid function tests so you can also monitor your progress. You can also log in there other things such as your weight or mood, as well as other factors that may either cause or be affected by your hyperthyroid condition. It is also wise to jot down any changes that you notice on your body, especially on your symptoms, as these will help determine how your body reacts to the treatments you are undergoing. This will help your physician decide whether or not you have to adjust your dosages, change your medications, or try a different type of treatment.

4. If you have Graves' ophthalmopathy, a condition in which the muscles in your eyes may swell, it can be helpful to use eye drops to help keep your eyes moist. Use protective eye wears such as sunglasses, especially when going out. It is also important to wear eye patches or use a clean cloth or gauze to cover your eyes before sleeping; this condition can cause your eyes to remain partially open even as you sleep, and leaving your eyes exposed can get them permanently damaged. Make sure to consult an ophthalmologist as he will

recommend eye drops and/or ointments to help make sure that the condition doesn't worsen.

5. Keep your head elevated, even when you sleep. This is to help reduce the swelling and the pressure on your eyes.

6. If you have Graves' dermopathy, or a swelling of the skin, you may apply over-the-counter creams for swollen skin, particularly creams with hydrocortisone. Use this to relieve the swollen skin of your feet or shins. You may have your doctor give you a prescription or simply inform you about these creams.

7. If your hyperthyroid condition is caused by thyroiditis, you can use an ice pack (or an ice cube wrapped in a clean cloth if you don't have one) and apply it to your throat area to help reduce the inflammation of your thyroid glands.

8. Shy away from cafés. Unfortunately for coffee lovers, caffeine can worsen many symptoms associated with hyperthyroidism, including an increased heart rate, difficulty in concentrating, and nervousness.

9. Quit smoking. This piece of advice may have been mentioned here several times already, but this is only because it is a very important one. It can worsen symptoms of your condition, and even cause you to develop other forms of thyroid problems that you don't already have. For instance, a person's Graves' disease might progress to Graves' ophthalmopathy if he smokes. Also avoid taking in second hand smoke as this can have the same effects even if you are a non-smoker.

10. Allow yourself at least an hour each day for de-stressing. Do anything simple that you know will allow you to relax your body and mind. It can be something as simple as listening to soothing music, or going to a quiet place and meditating there, or treating yourself to a long, relaxing bath.

11. Don't make any major dietary changes without first consulting with your endocrinologist and a licensed dietitian.

12. Incorporate regular exercise into your lifestyle changes. Even a good diet isn't much help without physical activity. This doesn't have to be anything that is too time-consuming, expensive, or strenuous. Simple activities like walking, dancing, or gardening will already count as good physical activities.

13. Drink lots and lots of water to help cleanse the body of toxins and also regulate the absorption of key nutrients from the food you take. It is advisable to drink at least 2 liters of water daily.

14. Maintain a positive outlook and try to keep yourself happy. Depression is often associated as a symptom for hypothyroidism and not hyperthyroidism. However, it is still possible for a hyperthyroid patient to experience depression due to some of the more problematic symptoms that come with their disease. For instance, many people with Graves' ophthalmopathy often feel a sudden sense of insecurity because of their bulging eyes, which can lead

to depression. Do not hesitate to seek professional help, as major emotional and psychological stress that is caused by depression can only worsen your condition.

15. You can search for support groups that can help you in managing hyperthyroidism. There are some support groups that are composed of individuals with the same condition. It is much easier to go through the necessary lifestyle changes if there are other people around you who can understand what you are going through. You will also be able to pick up some other helpful tips from them to make it easier for you to live through your condition.

Always remember that you are always stronger than your diseases. You shouldn't let your condition control you; rather, you should be the one controlling your condition. The fact that you may have hyperthyroidism doesn't mean that you're going to have to stop eating the foods you love or doing things that you enjoy. You can still go on with your life and live it normally despite your thyroid disease. It is all a matter of maintaining balance: the right medications, proper nutrition from a healthy diet, regular physical activity, and a happy and positive disposition.

Conclusion

Thank you again for purchasing this book!

I hope this book was able to help you to differentiate the different medical conditions which may have some sort of connection to hyperthyroidism. I hope that by reading this eBook, you will be better off equipped with medical knowledge that you can impart or share with those you love who apparently are suffering the same fate.

Your new-found learning about hyperthyroidism will greatly help you in overcoming the negative effects of this condition and you can certainly help out in making sure that medications are properly administered to the patient.

The next step is to share this information with the people you love. You can also inspire others to read this eBook so that they, too can learn what you have learned.

Finally, if you enjoyed this book, please take the time to share your thoughts and post a review on Amazon. We do our best to reach out to readers and provide the best value we can. Your positive review will help us achieve that. It'd be greatly appreciated!

Thank you and good luck!

Check Out My Other Books

Below you'll find some of my other popular books that are popular on Amazon and Kindle as well. Simply click on the links below to check them out. Alternatively, you can visit my author page on Amazon to see other work done by me.

Coconut Oil for Easy Weight Loss

http://amzn.to/1i5f45p

Essential Oils & Aromatherapy

http://amzn.to/1ouuZTx

Carrier Oils For Beginners

http://amzn.to/1sbqUQP

Natural Homemade Cleaning Recipes For Beginners

http://amzn.to/1izDB2m

Superfoods that Kickstart Your Weight Loss

http://amzn.to/1eyHdku

The Best Secrets Of Natural Remedies

http://amzn.to/1gmHd7y

The Hypothyroidism Handbook

http://amzn.to/1emWfyR

The Hyperthyroidism Handbook

http://amzn.to/1kqLQCp

Essential Oils & Weight Loss For Beginners
http://amzn.to/Q83bFp

Top Essential Oil Recipes
http://amzn.to/1lSrhSC

Soap Making For Beginners
http://amzn.to/1fkmYwr

Body Butters For Beginners
http://amzn.to/1fWjwJe

Apple Cider Vinegar For Beginners
http://amzn.to/1joDzX2

Homemade Body Scrubs & Masks For Beginners
http://amzn.to/1jjLRIO

The Beginners Guide To Medicinal Plants
http://amzn.to/1vSujr6

The Beginners Guide To Making Your Own Essential Oils
http://amzn.to/1piUNSB

The Beginners Alkaline Miracle Diet
http://amzn.to/1sDVaVE

Thyroid Diet
http://amzn.to/1piW2RY

Essential Oils Box Set #1 (Weight Loss + Essential Oil Recipes
http://amzn.to/1qlYWWP

Essential Oils Box Set #2 (Weight Loss + Essential Oil & Aromatherapy
http://amzn.to/1qlYWWP

Essential Oils Box Set #3 Coconut Oil + Apple Cider Vinegar
http://amzn.to/1oIFZJw

Essential Oils Box Set #4 Body Butters & Top Essential Oil Recipes
http://amzn.to/1jSxURJ

Essential Oils Box Set #5 Soap Making & Homemade Body Scrubs
http://amzn.to/RAvJYo

Essential Oils Box Set #6 Body Butters & Body Scrubs
http://amzn.to/RAvSel

Essential Oils Box Set #7 Top Essential Oils & Best Kept Secrets Of Natural Remedies
http://amzn.to/1gvsRCq

Essential Oils Box Set #8 Homemade Cleaning Recipes & Essential Oil Recipes

http://amzn.to/1gxFAVb

Essential Oils Box Set #9 Essential Oil and Weight Loss & Carrier Oils

http://amzn.to/1jmcEPP

Essential Oils Box Set #10 Hyperthyroidism Manual & Hypothyroidism Manual

http://amzn.to/1nHgJU4

Essential Oils Box Set #11 Carrier Oils for Beginners & Coconut Oil for Easy Weight Loss

http://amzn.to/1nHfy6X

Essential Oils Box Set #12 Essential Oils Weight Loss & Essential Oils Aromatherapy & Natural Homemade Cleaning Supplies & Top Essential Oil Recipes & Carrier Oils

http://amzn.to/1nHfy6X

Essential Oils Box Set #13 Superfoods & Essential Weight Loss & Essential Aromatherapy & Body Butters & Soap Making

http://amzn.to/1nUds6v

Essential Oils Box Set #14 Weight Loss & Apple Cider Vinegar & Body Butters & Homemade Body Scrubs & Coconut Oil for Beginners

http://amzn.to/1i1qYOd

If the links do not work, for whatever reason, you can simply search for these titles on the Amazon website to find them.

www.ingramcontent.com/pod-product-compliance
Lightning Source LLC
Chambersburg PA
CBHW070721180526
45167CB00004B/1572